This book belongs to:

An Incredible Person!

Printed in the United States of America

First Printing, 2015

ISBN 978-1-943880-00-3
Library of Congress Control Number 2015947226

BlueFox Press
Saratoga Springs, UT 84045

BlueFoxPress.com

Millie the Cat has Borderline Personality Disorder

by jessie shepherd, ACMHC   illustrations ty shepherd

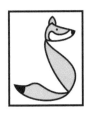

an imprint of
BlueFox Press

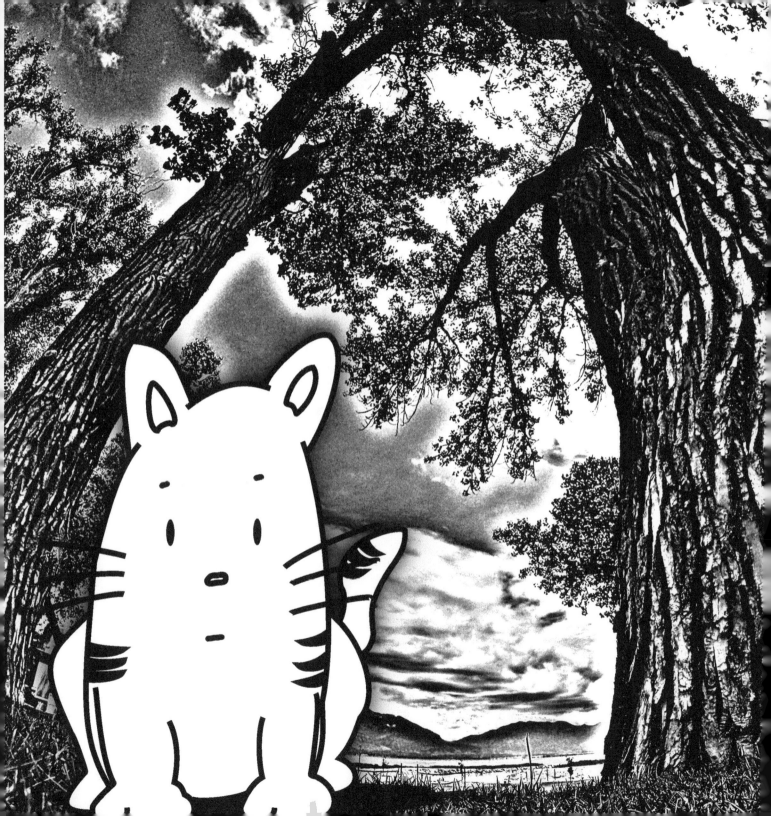

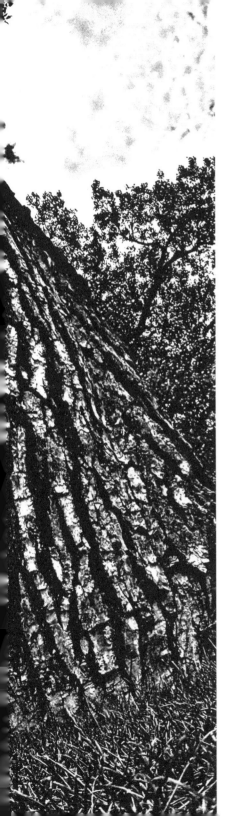

This is Millie. She has
Borderline Personality Disorder.

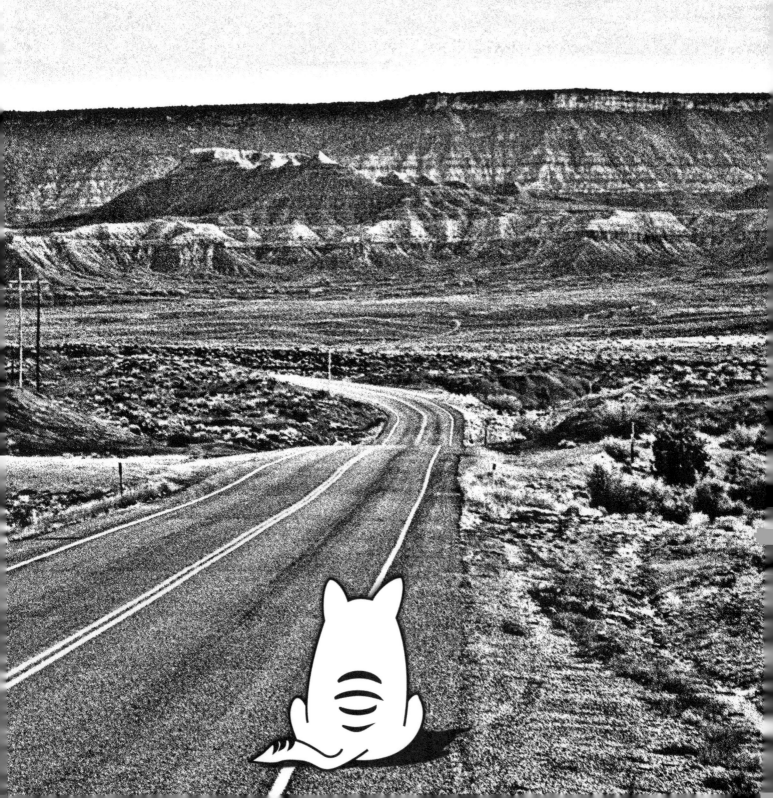

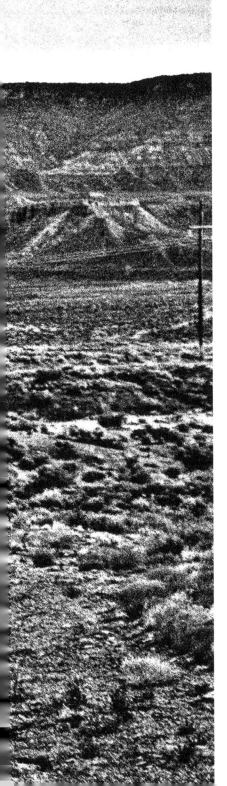

She is scared of being alone.

She hates being alone.

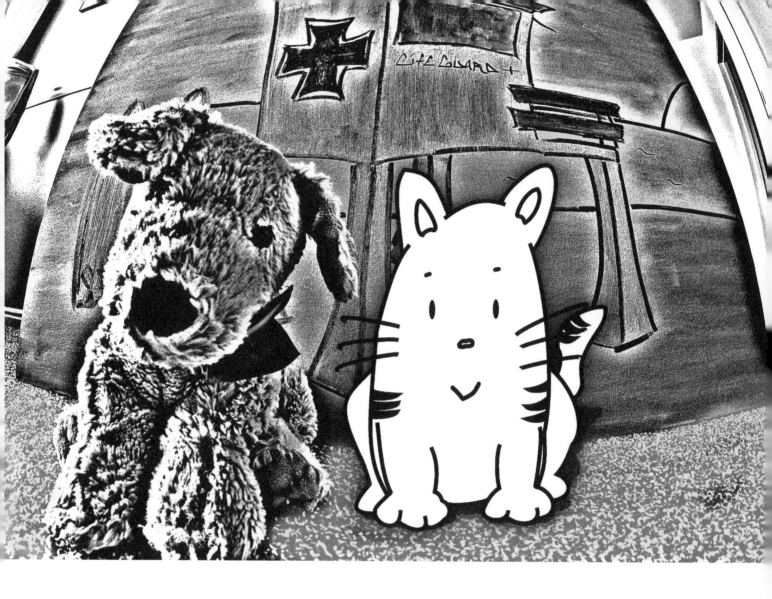

Sometimes she sees her friend Peter as
completely perfect.

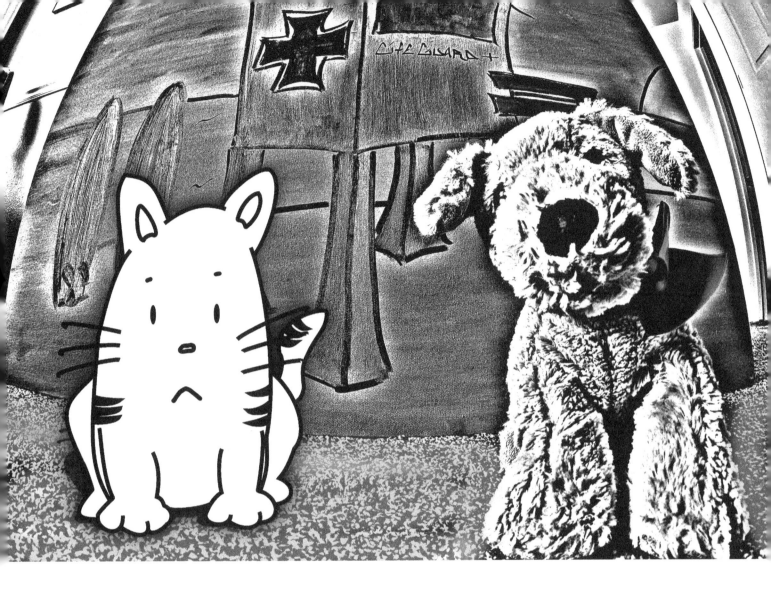

Sometimes she sees Peter as all bad.

Either way she does not want
him to leave.

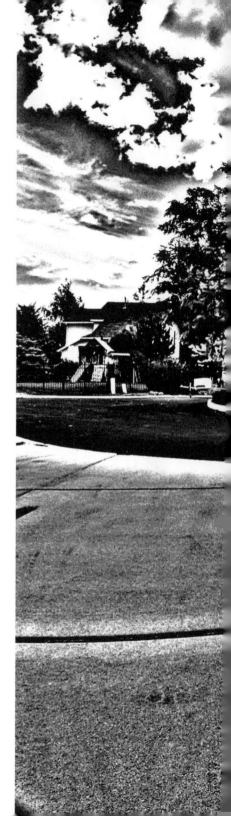

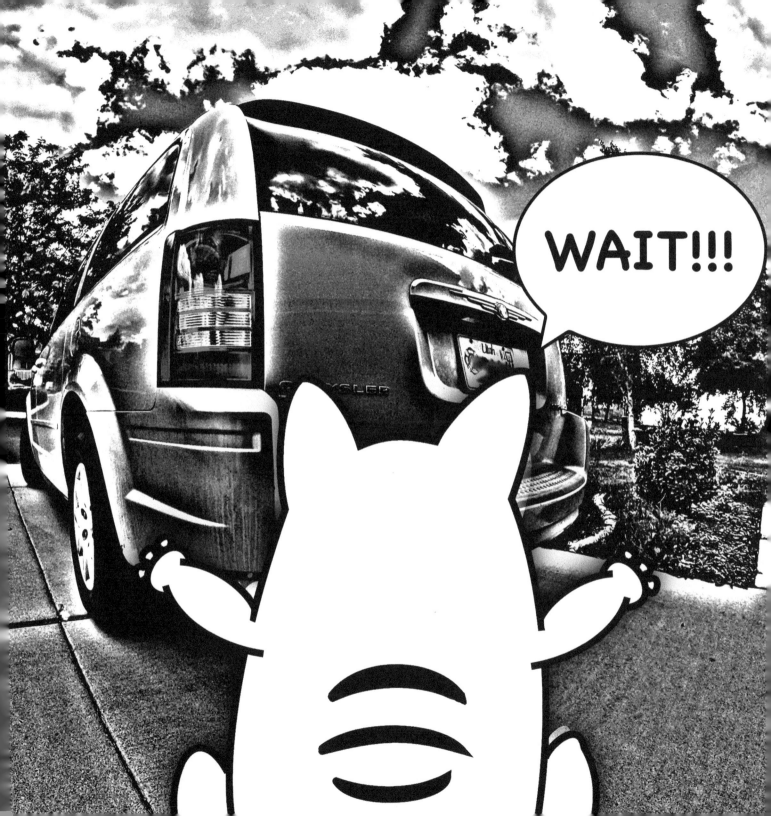

Sometimes Millie has intense anger.

Which makes her feel guilty.

Which makes her feel worthless.

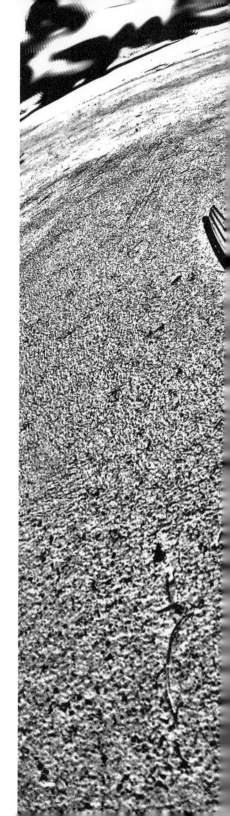

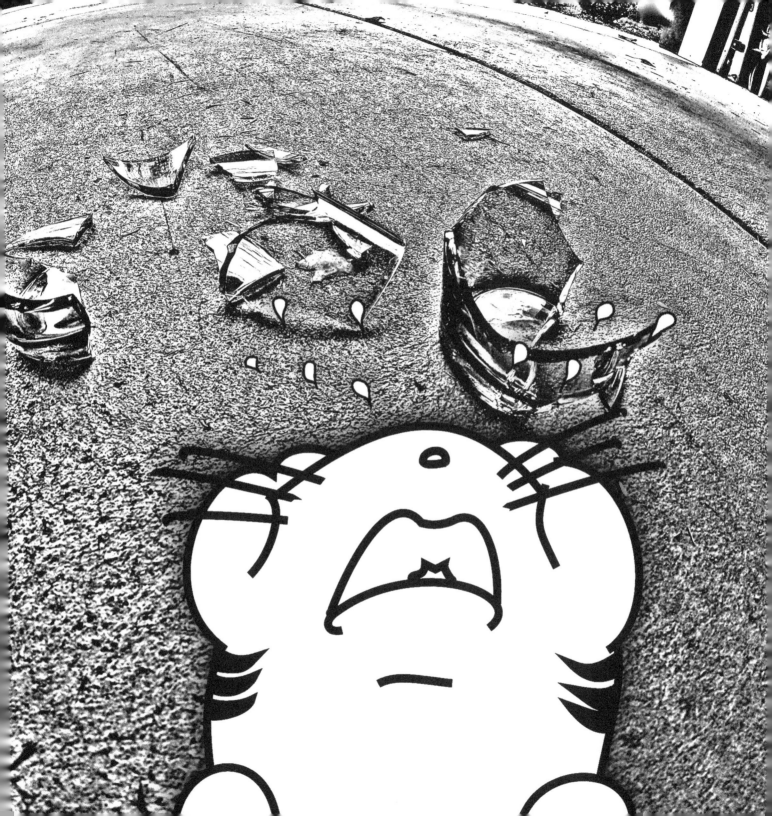

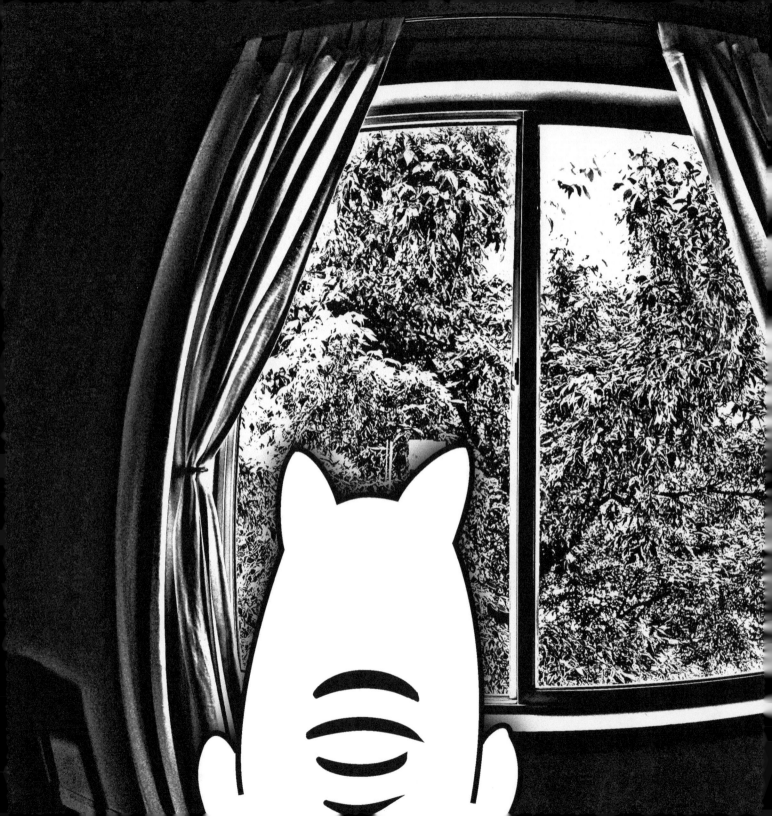

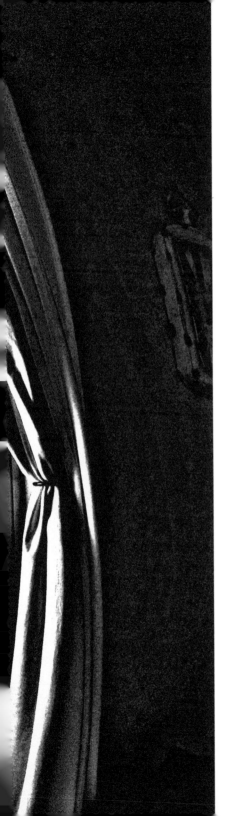

Sometimes people don't want to hang out with Millie because of her anger.

This makes Millie feel like she is not wanted.

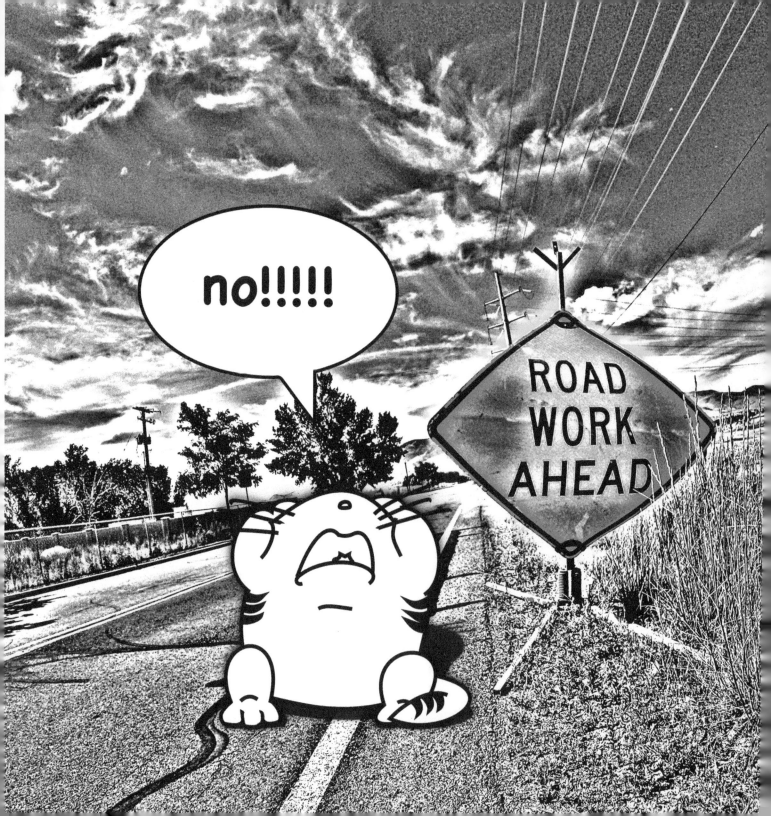

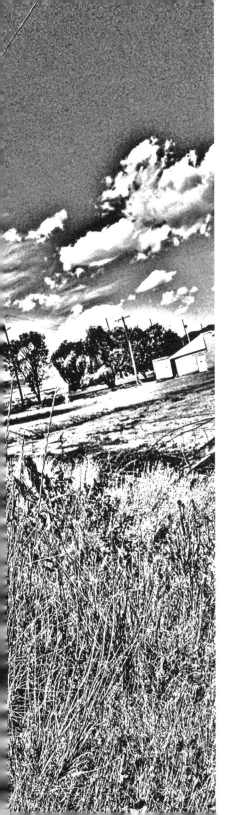

Millie does not like when she can't control change.

She tends to panic if someone is not on time, even if they have a good reason.

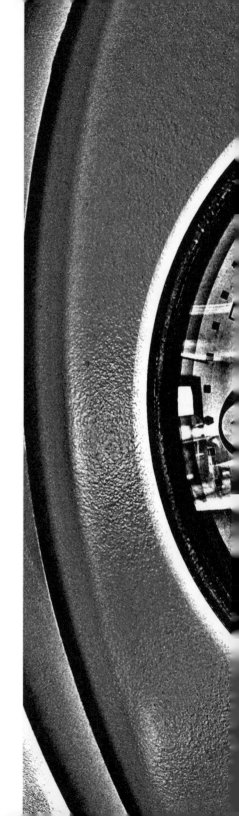

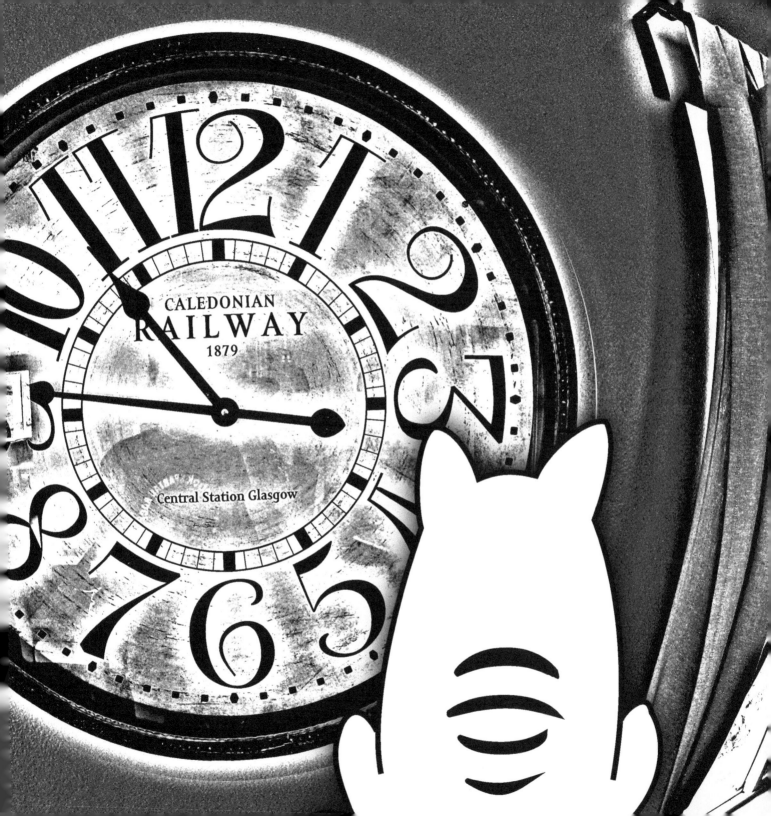

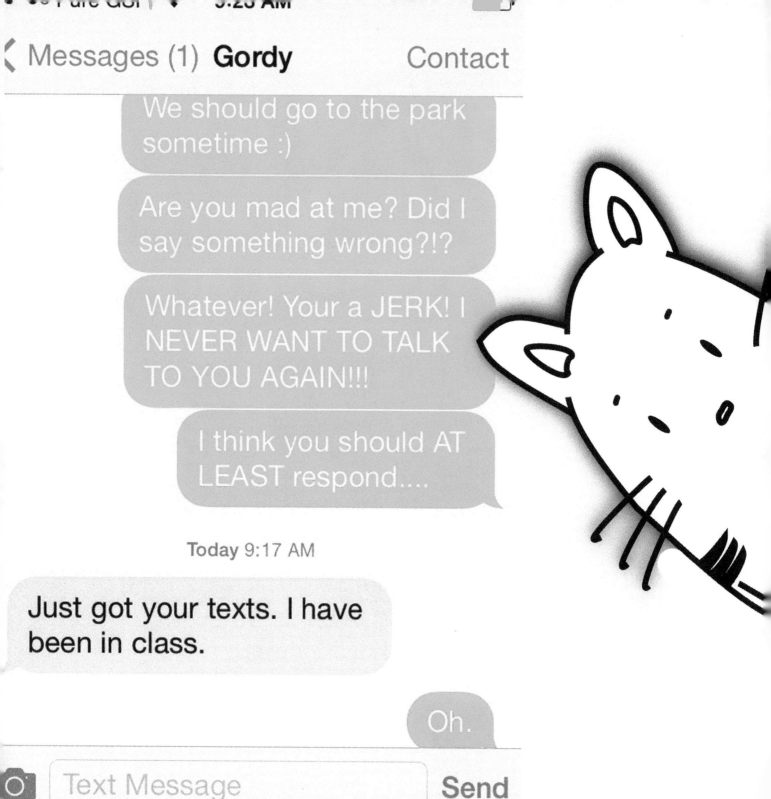

She has frantic behaviors like texting or calling over and over to keep people from leaving her.

This just makes things worse.

Sometimes Millie feels so empty she does not want to exist anymore.

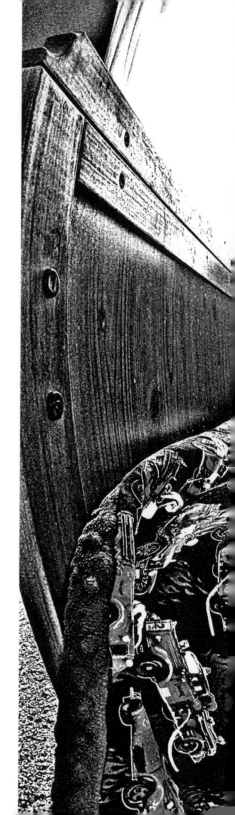

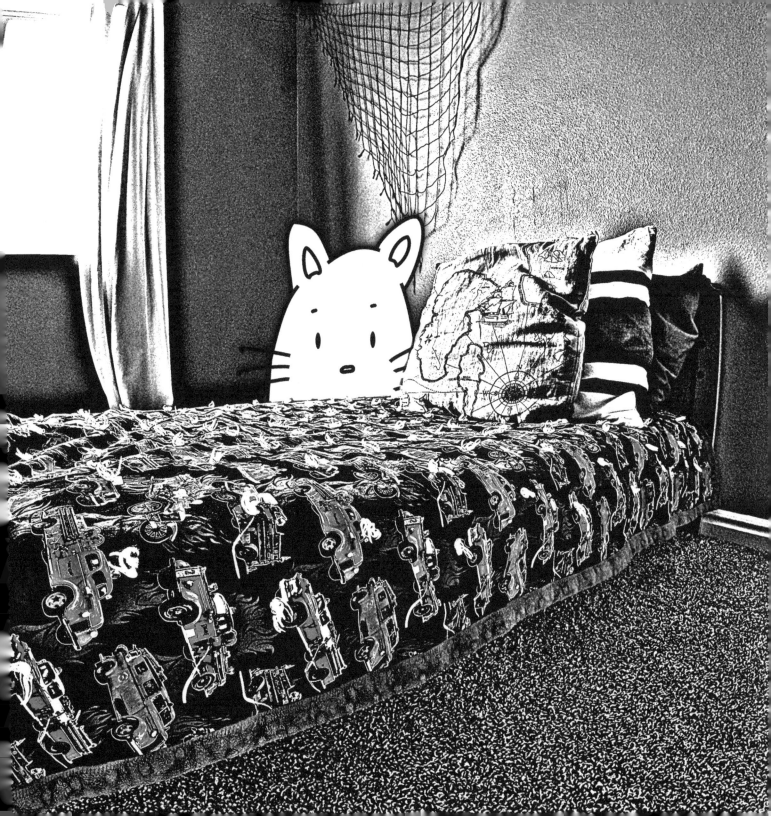

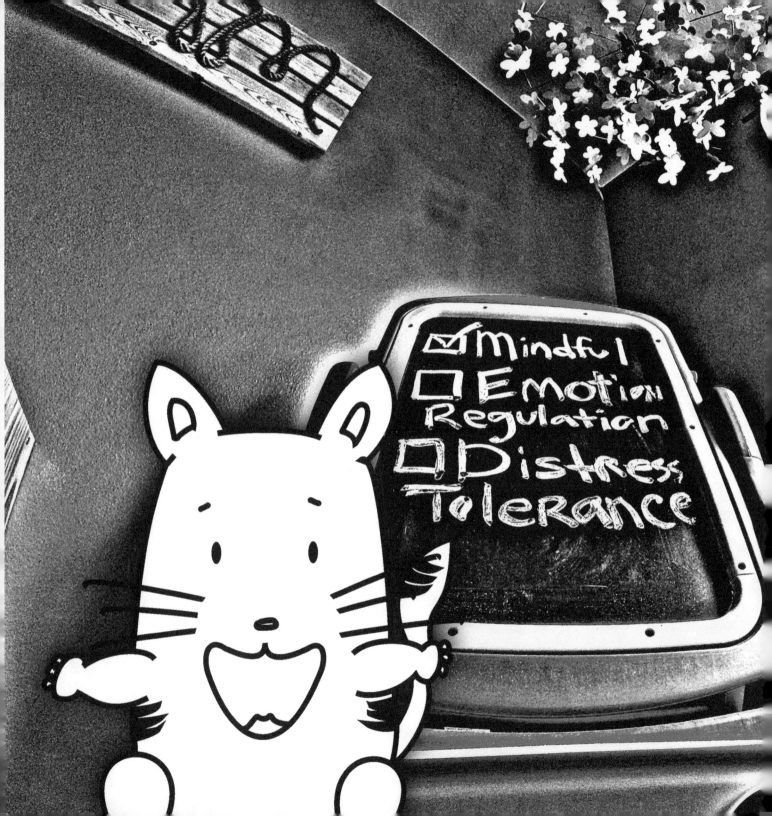

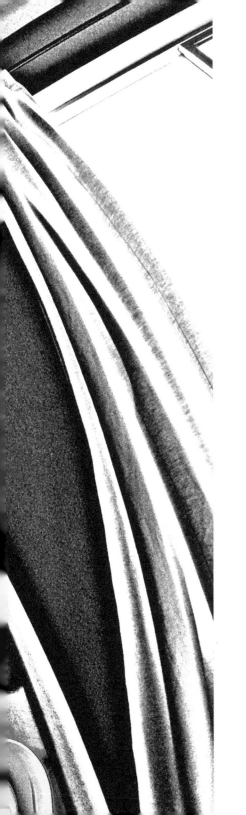

But there is hope for Millie.

She can learn skills to feel better.

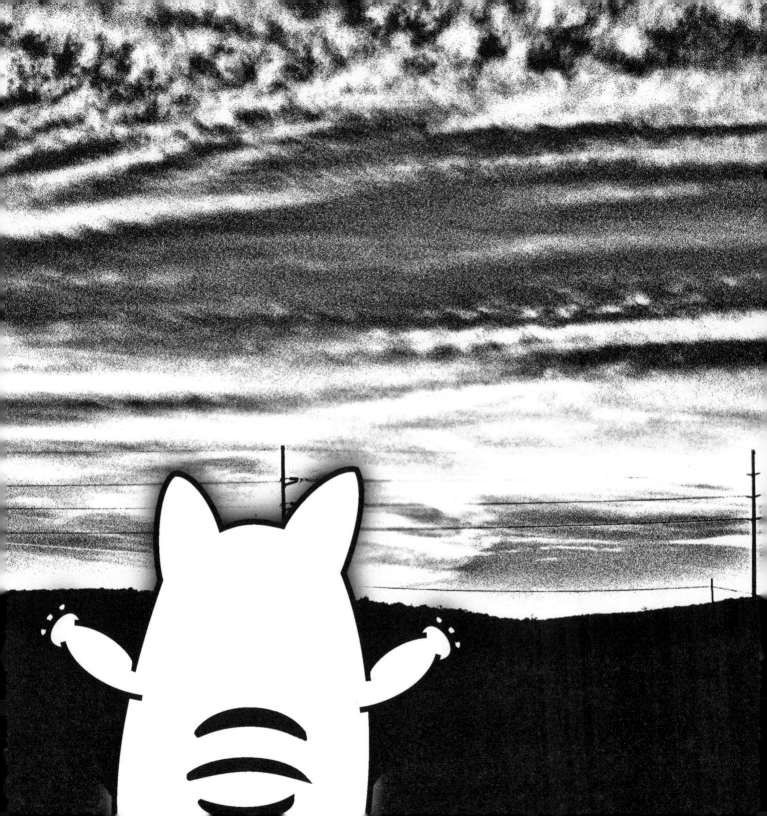

Like being in the moment and thinking things through.

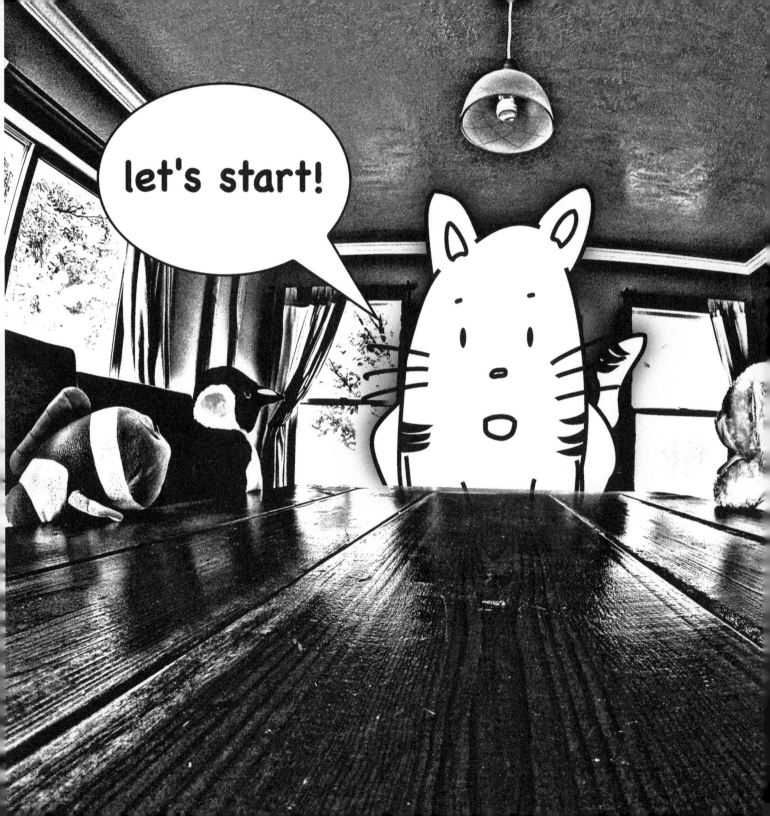

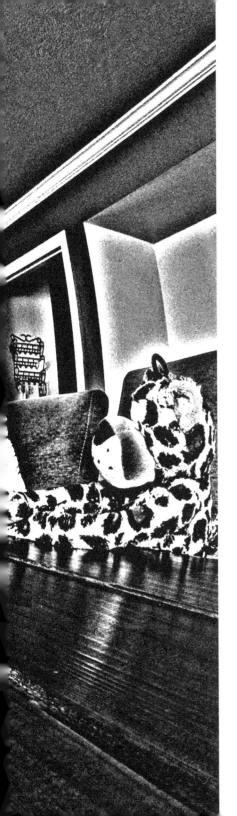

Or expressing what she feels
while staying calm and
confident.

Plus some amazing things come from having Borderline Personality Disorder.

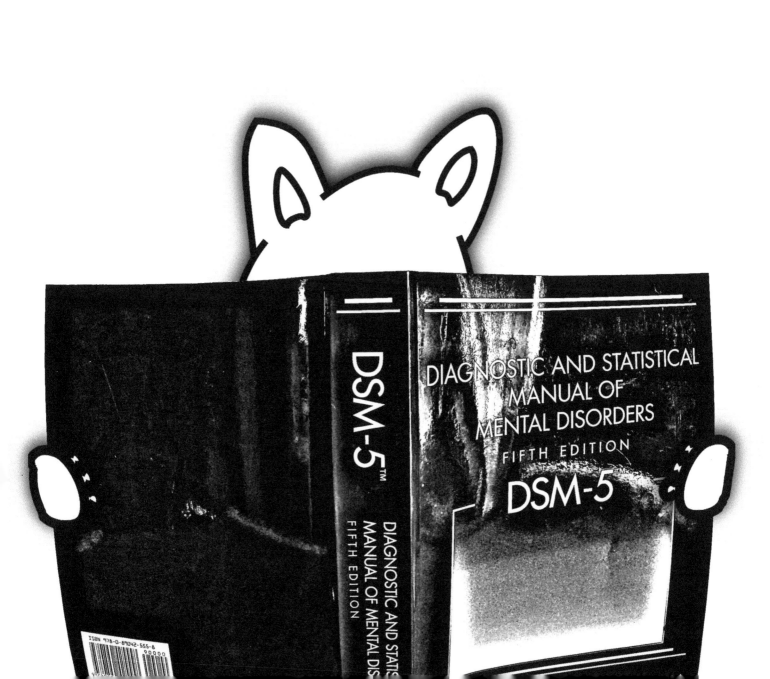

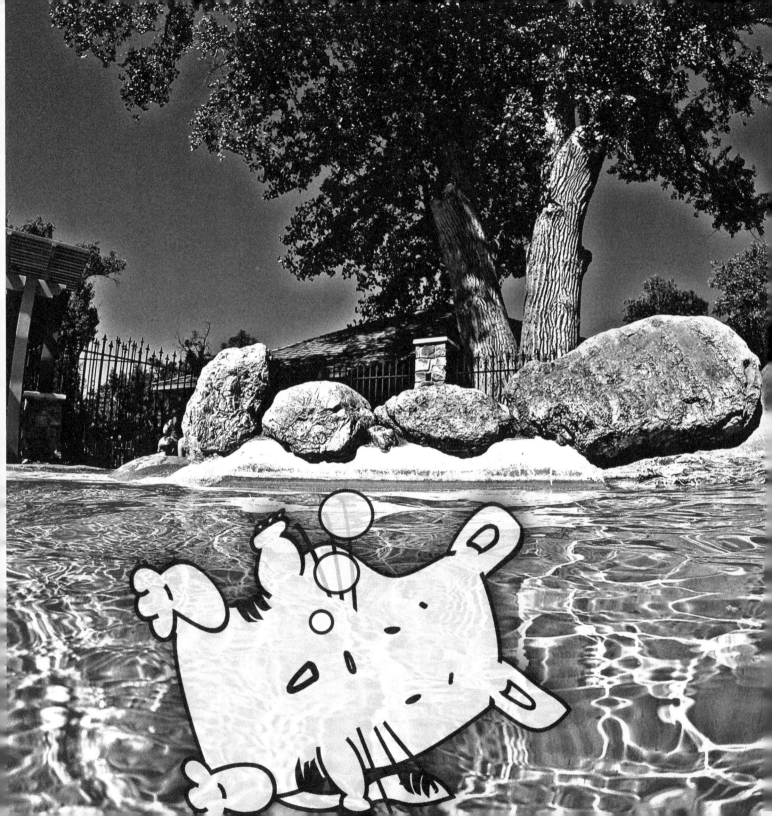

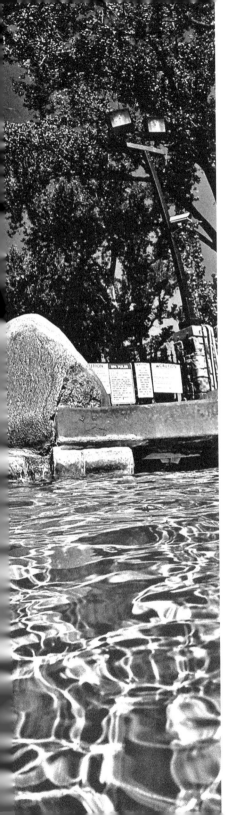

Like how she feels
emotions so deep.

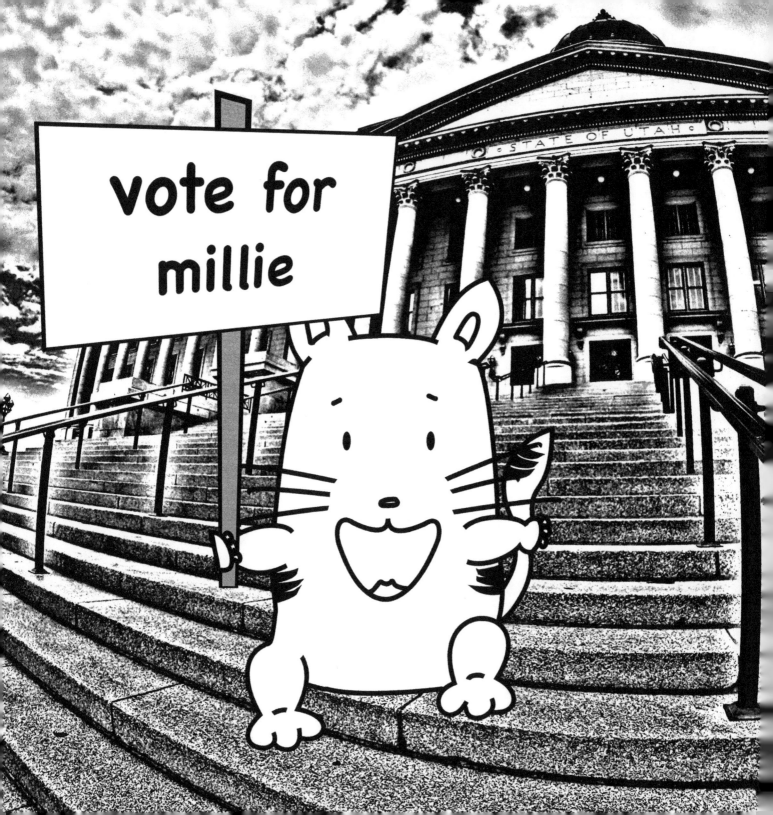

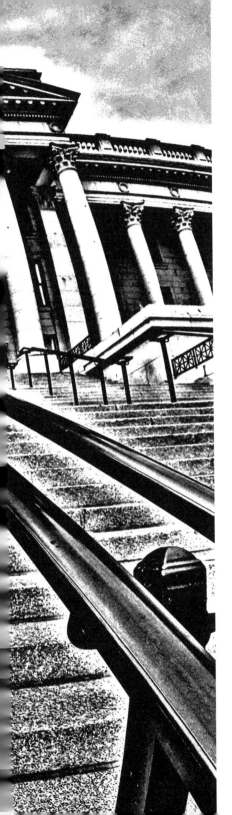

This makes her passionate about causes she cares for, so she works extra hard for them.

It also fuels creativity for music, painting, writing poetry, dancing and acting.

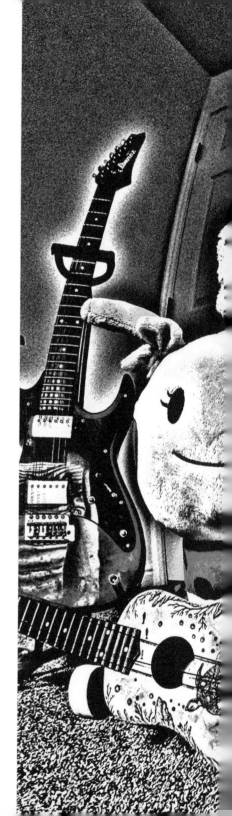

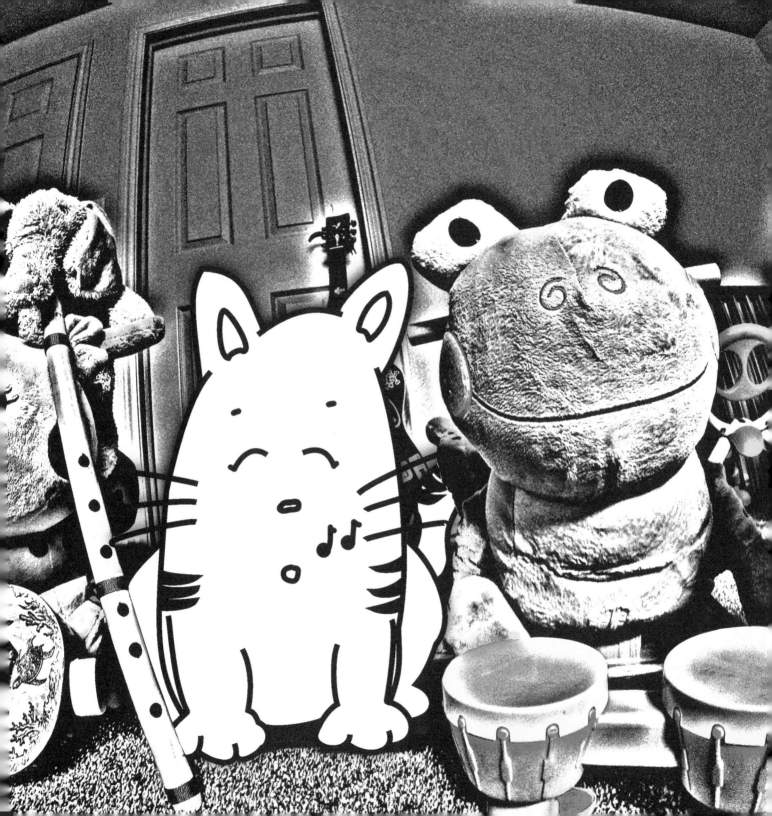

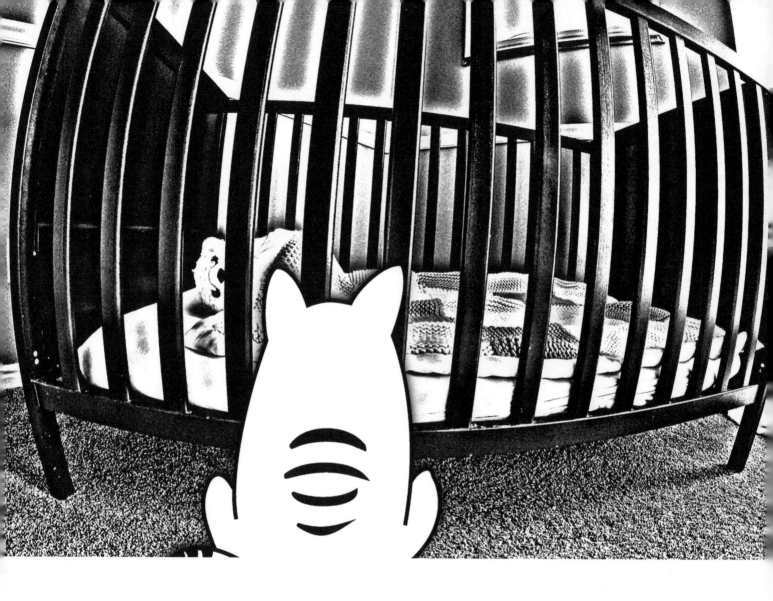

She is an excellent helper and caretaker.

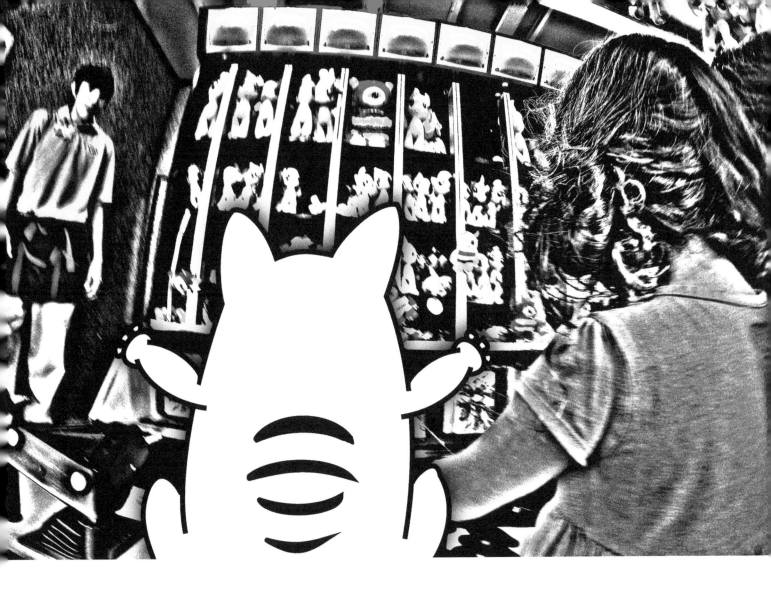

She cares so much she can pick up on what others need to feel better.

She even sees aspects in others that
most people miss.

Like when people try to hide that they
are hurt or scared.

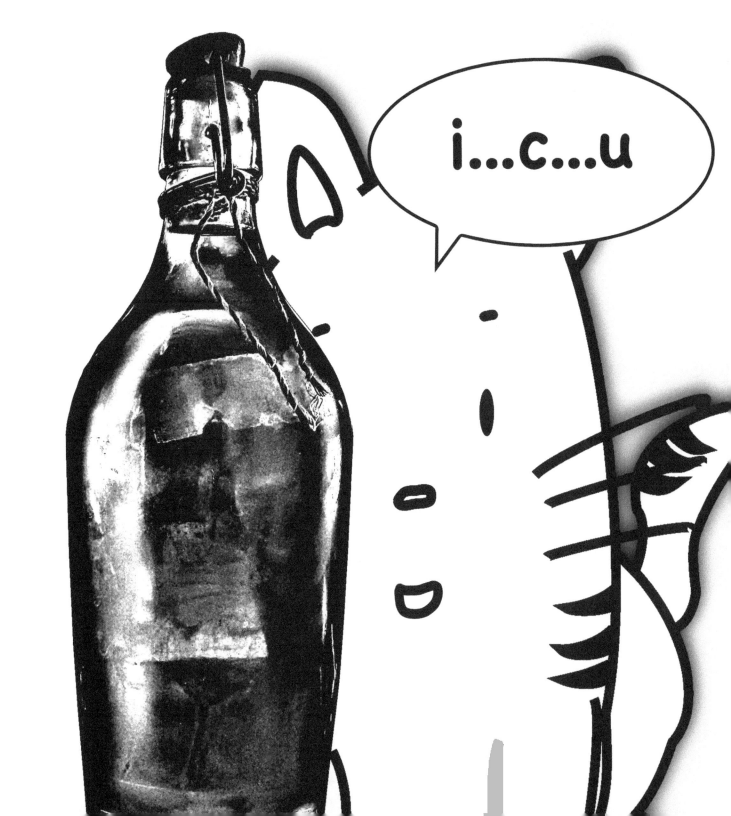

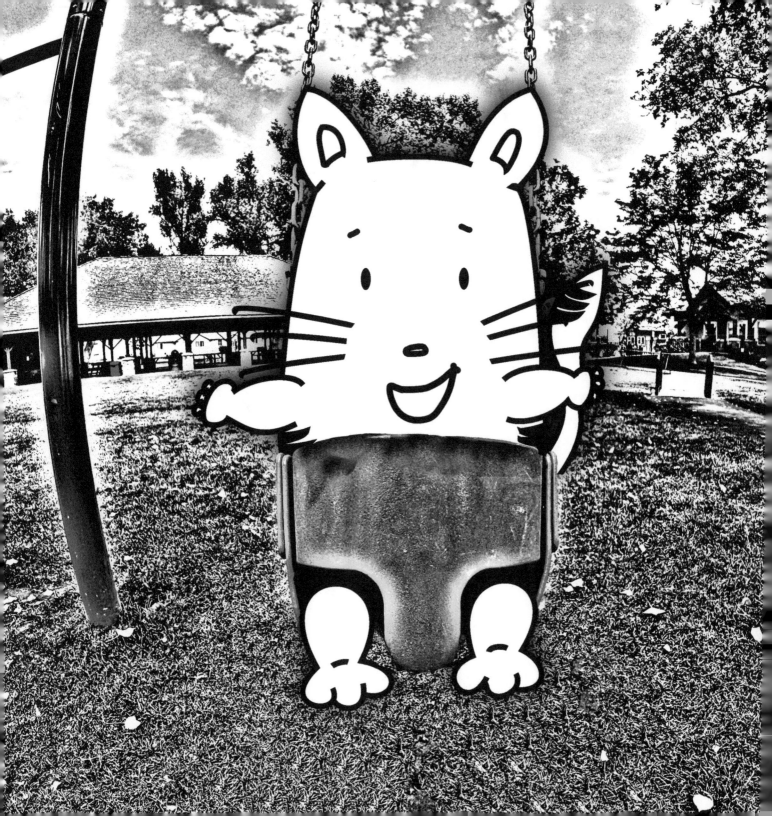

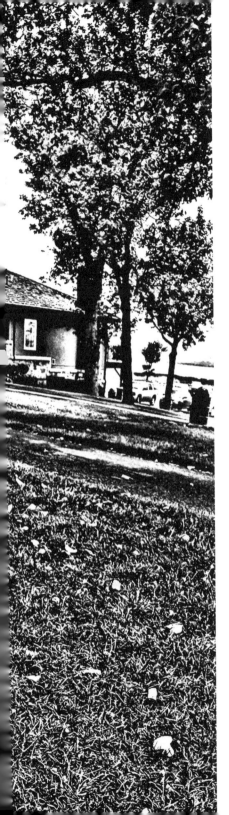

She is very adventurous
and spontaneous.

She can adapt to new situations quickly and make them way more fun.

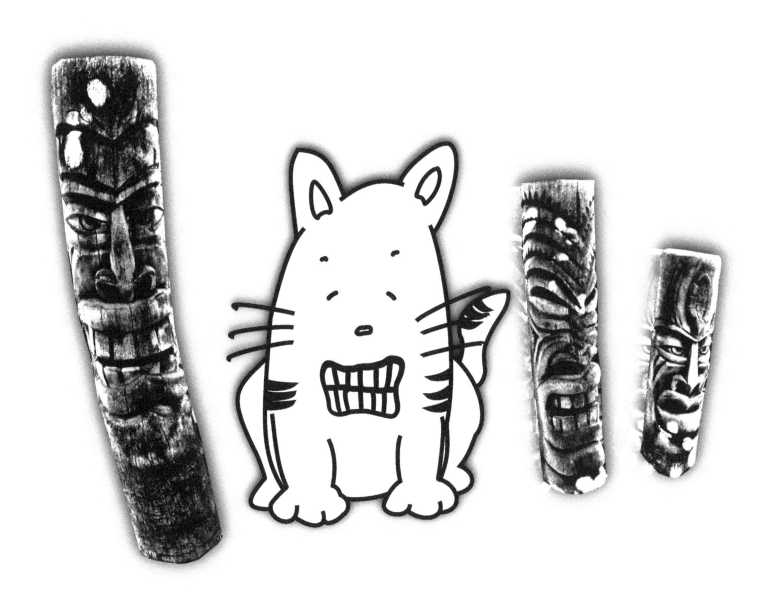

Millie is also strong and brave which makes her able to achieve anything she puts her mind to!

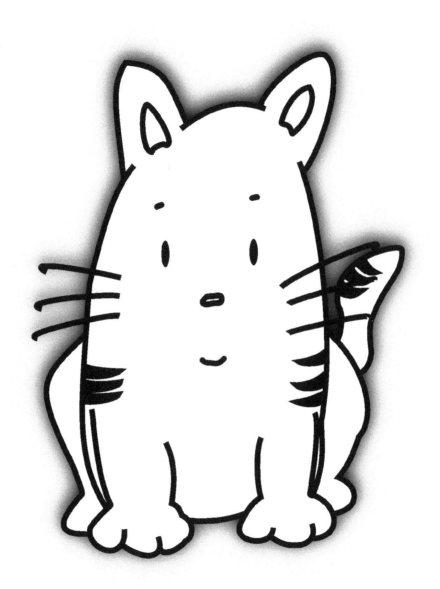

Best way to interact with someone with Borderline Personality Disorder

-They do well with structure, so holding to rules and boundaries is very important.

-Stick with the facts, don't get caught up in the emotion.

-Everyone in the family needs to learn distress tolerance, mindfulness and emotional regulation skills in order to help each other use them.

-Continue with therapy knowing that it is a lot of work but will be helpful for your whole life.

-Understand that skill building is a process and no one will be perfect instantly.

-Have patience with each other.

-Seek professional support for you and your family. Dialectic Behavioral Therapy is one of the leading therapies shown to be effective treatment for Borderline Personality Disorder.

CPSIA information can be obtained
at www.ICGtesting.com
Printed in the USA
LVHW072103010422
714606LV00037B/1044